I0414982

The Educated Eating Manual

Also by Chris Barrows
The Feeling Of Fit

Visit the website for news and updates:
www.TheFeelingOfFit.com

The Educated Eating Manual

by
Chris Barrows

Cover Artwork:
Tom Roach

Edited by:
Cheryl Connell

Photos & Layout:
Leif Quitevis

iUniverse, Inc.
New York Bloomington

The Educated Eating Manual

Copyright © 2010 by Chris Barrows

All rights reserved. No part of this book may be used or reproduced by any means, graphic, electronic, or mechanical, including photocopying, recording, taping or by any information storage retrieval system without the written permission of the publisher except in the case of brief quotations embodied in critical articles and reviews.

You should not undertake any diet/exercise regimen recommended in this book before consulting your personal physician. Neither the author nor the publisher shall be responsible or liable for any loss or damage allegedly arising as a consequence of your use or application of any information or suggestions contained in this book.

iUniverse books may be ordered through booksellers or by contacting:

iUniverse
1663 Liberty Drive
Bloomington, IN 47403
www.iuniverse.com
1-800-Authors (1-800-288-4677)

Because of the dynamic nature of the Internet, any Web addresses or links contained in this book may have changed since publication and may no longer be valid. The views expressed in this work are solely those of the author and do not necessarily reflect the views of the publisher, and the publisher hereby disclaims any responsibility for them.

ISBN: 978-1-4502-3620-1 (sc)
ISBN: 978-1-4502-3631-7 (ebook)

Printed in the United States of America

iUniverse rev. date: 06/03/2010

*This book is dedicated to the city
and people of Corpus Christi TX,
a magical town where dreams can come true.*

Preface

Our bodies are made up of the food we eat. Foods we consume dictate how our body will perform. In this book you will find foods that will: increase your energy, help you lose weight, help you focus, increase your strength, be a better lover, help you live longer, and more. After reading this book, you will know how to improve your life with food.

Don't be fooled by false claims, get the facts. This fun and easy to read book contains the most recent information about the effects that foods and drinks have on the body. Will fruits or vegetables help you run faster? Will you gain more muscle mass consuming protein powders or whole foods? Will you live longer by eating fish?

You were given only one body; take care of it, and it will take care of you.

Acknowledgements

A special thanks goes to Jessica Pennington, Leif Quitevis, Dean Lucas, Jon Hueber, Eric Hanselmann, Carolyn Neal, and Jessica George for their help in transferring this book from a thought to a reality.

Using This Book

Thank you for picking up **The Educated Eating Manual**. This book was fun to write and I hope you enjoy it. The main point that I have to make before you begin is that this book is designed to help you choose foods that will help you toward a specific goal. However, the human body requires a variety of foods to enable it to function properly and give you the best performance.

The best guide in determining how much food to eat and from which specific group is the USDA food pyramid. Make sure to include a variety of foods daily. If you have specific nutritional needs, consult your doctor before making any changes.

With each page containing separate subjects, this book is meant for you to be able to skip around and find the subject that fits your goals. Yes, you made the right, educated decision by choosing **The Educated Eating Manual**.

Table of Contents

Introduction

Our bodies are in tune with nature. We are affected by what happens around us. If it is rainy day, we feel and act differently than if it were a sunny day. Other people or animals around us affect our moods. The food we eat and liquids we drink also affect how we look, act, and feel.

We all know asparagus makes your pee smell funny, and that coffee wakes you up, but most people don't know how other foods affect the body. Common knowledge will tell you that eating healthy food is good for you, but many do not know that what they eat affects their mood, immunity, energy levels, sex drive, focus, and life span.

This book will show you how to become more in tune with your body and with nature. Being educated on what the foods you put into your body are doing, or not doing, will help you perform the way you want to perform, and live a long, healthy life.

Learn what foods and drinks will help you sleep better, grow your hair, clean your body, keep vital organs healthy, improve your eyesight, and adjust your weight.

Don't underestimate the importance of food and drink, without it we would be dead. We are what we eat, and what you put in your mouth makes you who you are.

How Food Began

In early times, even before fast food, Man found that the rumbling in his stomach meant that he should find something to put in it. When he found something that he could sink his teeth through - and if it tasted halfway decent - he ate it, and it settled the feeling in his stomach. If he lived the next day, he ate it again. They had a very simple rule back then: if the person eating the food before you holds their throat, gasps for air, and falls over dead, you didn't eat the same thing that they did. Experimenting with new foods was a little more intense in those days.

Today, we can feel confident that the foods we pick off the shelves at the grocery store are safe to eat. The trial and error part of finding safe and edible foods is over.

Some of the foods we eat were discovered by accident. Corn flakes and potato chips were discovered inadvertently. The invention of the microwave oven was discovered by mistake as well. Many recipes have been made by someone adding a wrong ingredient, or trying something new, and after tasting their creation, they had come up with a better recipe.

Thank your early ancestors for the food you eat today. Somebody at sometime had to be the first one to try the foods you eat. Back then, finding which foods contain health benefits could take generations to determine. Now we have science to help us determine which food benefits the body.

Water

I am going to start this book by stressing the importance of water. Every living thing on the planet depends on water to survive; your body is no exception. Your body has many systems and organs that would not last very long without water. Sodas and sports drinks are no substitute for water. Many drinks with alcohol or caffeine can even dehydrate you even more.

Somewhere, somebody said that you need eight glasses of water a day. Well, that is minimum for a non-active person. There are many other variables that require you to drink more than eight glasses of water per day. Exercising regularly, working in the heat, eating salty foods, and drinking alcohol all increase your body's requirement for water.

The body uses water to: cool down, keep organs functioning, flush out toxins, and to transport oxygen just to name a few purposes. Food only provides ten percent of needed water intake. If your urine is bright yellow, you are dehydrated.

Eat To Live Longer

To live a long, healthy life is the desire of most people. One of the most important things you can do to ensure that your life will not be cut short due to illness or disease is to eat right. Eating balanced meals will provide your body with the nutrients it needs to function properly.

There are other ways to extend your life expectancy, and help your body to live longer. One way is not to overeat. Eat less and live longer. Many studies have concluded that people, within their correct weight limits, will live longer than those who are overweight. So think twice before taking that second helping, you might be cutting time off your life.

There are certain foods that can help you extend your life as well. Here are some suggestions for those who want to live a longer life; eat fruits, vegetables, fish, and don't step in front of any moving vehicles. Fish, with its omega 3 fatty acids, can help reduce premature aging. Fruits and vegetables will keep your systems healthy, strawberries in particular can protect against age related diseases. Green tea and blueberries have powerful antioxidants that keep your cardiovascular system healthy. Make sure to avoid stepping in front of moving vehicles as this can greatly reduce your life expectancy.

Sickness Fighting Foods

There are foods that help your body to fight off intruders that cause you to feel sick. Consuming these foods on a regular basis will help your immune system do the job of keeping you healthy.

Let's start off with fruit; bananas, berries, grapefruit, and other citrus fruit help to build immunity. Other helpful plant life includes: mushrooms, sweet potatoes, broccoli, spinach, beans, nuts, and whole grains.

Yogurt's live cultures act as little immune system fighters. Spices such as: ginger, garlic, honey, and cinnamon help in the fight against sickness.

If you are already sick, there are a few foods that will help provide fast relief for your symptoms. Many people had their mom make them chicken soup when they were sick. Moms know best, chicken soup and plenty of clear fluids like water and tea will help to get you back on your feet. Eating about 20 tart cherries could reduce inflammatory pain and headache pain. Spicy foods and chilies can clear your congestion.

Consuming foods that have no nutritional value will most likely taste great, but sooner or later your body's defenses will break down from lack of proper nutrients, and you will get sick. If that pastry or greasy burger is worth it, and you end up getting sick, don't come crying to me. Try crying to your mom, maybe she will make you some chicken soup.

Disease Fighting Foods

Having good genes is one of the major factors that determine your chances of avoiding a disease. Experts also agree that watching what you eat can increase your body's ability to protect itself, and lower your chances of contracting cancer or disease.

The following foods help your body fight against cancer: onions, garlic, lemons, tomatoes, flaxseeds, mushrooms, whole grains, dark leafy greens, pumpkin seeds, soy, berries, carrots, and coconut. Beans and other legumes have been shown to reduce colon cancer. Cooked tomatoes help to fight prostate cancer. Cabbage helps to reduce breast and many other kinds of cancers, and blueberries will fight all kinds of cancers.

These foods help fight against cardiovascular disease: garlic, berries, cherries, fruits, spinach, carrots, sweet potatoes, vegetables, whole grains, and fish. Other ways to help reduce your risk of developing heart disease is by drinking enough water, lowering sodium intake, and watching your saturated fat consumption.

Incorporating any one or more than one of these foods into your meals will help you avoid these diseases. Both cancer and cardiovascular disease have been allowed to run rampant too long and have taken far too many people. Until a cure is available, use these foods to reduce your chances of disease. If you like a person or a group of people, and you don't know how to say it to them, prepare some of these foods for them, and let the food tell them you want to see them stay around a while.

Brain Foods

Your brain does so many nice things for you, like helping you get out of bed in the morning, helping you decide what to wear, and what you are going to do, you should reward it by treating yourself to foods that will give you brain nurturing nutrients.

Here is a list of foods that help improve brain activity and memory. Making the top of the list is water. Always drink plenty of water, as dehydration will impair brain function. Fish, nuts, eggs, beans, and tofu help the brain. Fruits and vegetables also provide beneficial nutrients, along with raisin bran, sweet potatoes, beets and carrots. Berries like acai and blueberries contain brain-boosting qualities. Quite literally, you would be dumb not to eat these foods

Even dumber would be to abuse alcohol or illegal substances that damage the brain. The brain can actually repair damaged cells, but over time, the damaging effects of drugs and alcohol can be non-reversible. Stress can also have very negative effects on the health of the brain. Nutritious foods and regular exercise can help reverse the effects that stress can cause.

More food for thought; spinach, strawberries, and egg yolks can help fight some forms of brain disease. Next time you have to study for a test, it should be a no-brainer on which foods to eat.

Foods For Energy

We eat foods to provide our bodies with fuel to get us through our daily tasks and activities. Eating the right foods will provide us with sustained and efficient energy.

Apples, berries, and fresh fruit and juices are breakfast foods that give the most stamina with the least amount of calories. Nuts, seeds, oats, and whole grains are high, long lasting forms of energy. Eggs, yogurt, and beans are high in energy and protein. Vegetables, like fruits, are the best low calorie energy sources.

For a quick, healthy boost of energy, grab a handful of raisins and unsalted nuts. The effects are not as immediate or strong as caffeine or sugar, but they will last longer and not drop off as sudden.

In today's busy lifestyle, the immediate gratification of caffeine and sugar is widely recognized as the method for waking up and keeping pace with daily tasks. The proper food choices can do the same job. With heart related deaths ranking as the top killer, we need to make smarter choices. Switching to energy foods can help to wake you up, keep you going, and also relieve unnecessary stress on your ticker.

Depression Fighting Foods

Poor nutrition is a major cause of depression. Many years ago, it was found out that a lack of B vitamins caused depression symptoms, so manufacturers started fortifying products with B vitamins. That solution helped many people. Today, with our junk food trend and over caffeinated drinks, many foods lack nutrients, and it is no wonder that so many people suffer from depression symptoms. If your doctor did not ask about possible nutritional deficiencies in your eating habits before prescribing a depression pill, you might want to ask and find out if poor nutrition can be a cause of your symptoms.

Foods can pick you up when you are feeling down. These foods contain natural depression fighting nutrients: salmon, turkey, cabbage, milk, rice, pumpkin seeds, and whole grain oats. The nutritional contents in Brewer's yeast and cocoa can also help. Fruits and vegetables should always be chosen over foods that are high in fat. Taking a multivitamin will make sure your bases are covered.

Be careful, some known side effects from healthy eating include; healthy weight, increased confidence, increased energy, and a decrease in sickness. Also be careful when combining healthy eating with exercise and sunshine, as a healthy lifestyle may occur. In some cases, people have also displayed an increased tendency to smile and have fun.

Foods For Sex

Want to be a better lover? These foods help increase sexual performance and arousal. Raw oysters and figs top the list. Almonds, avocados, asparagus, bananas, eggs, nuts, fish, and of course, chocolate are all libido boosters. Other gender specific foods for stimulation are celery for women and oats for men.

Processed food, refined sugars, excess alcohol and caffeine all have a negative effect on sexual stamina. A consistent intake of the vitamins and nutrients found in fruits and vegetables can make it possible to increase blood flow and sexual stamina.

Spices to spice up your love life include pepper, ginger, clove, and basil. Regularly eating pineapple or drinking pineapple juice can potentially make oral sex for both men and women more pleasant. Onions, asparagus, and excess salt can negatively effect the enjoyment of oral sex. Watermelon contains ingredients that can possibly provide Viagra-like affects.

There is very little scientific research to back up these claims so you might want to do some research on your own to find what works best for you and your partner. You can explain to your partner that it is for the benefit of science.

Protein For Muscle Gain

There are many different types of muscle building products out there. These products come in many different forms, from protein bars to drinks and powders. Protein is also widely available in whole foods.

Some good whole food sources of protein are: soy, fish, beef, nuts, dairy, and beans. Your body uses protein for many different functions and purposes, but it can only use so much. If you eat more protein than your body needs, it is stored for energy or expelled as waste. An excessive intake of protein, over time, can have health risks. Your body needs a wide variety of foods for proper nourishment.

Your body needs protein to build and repair muscles after heavy usage. In my personal experience, I have not noticed a difference in either the whole food or the protein product method. If you find it easier and more convenient to grab a shake or a protein bar after a workout, then use this method to get your protein intake. Manufacturers keep making more convenient products. I think I have seen a product that had protein in chewing gum. It won't be long before you can download a picture of protein on your computer, and your muscles will get bigger just by looking at it.

Foods For Sleep, Hair, and Eyesight

Sleep

Foods that can help you get some sleep include bananas, oatmeal and warm milk. You can combine small amounts of all three together for a healthy alternative to a sleeping pill. There may not be any medical evidence to back up the claim that warm milk will help you sleep better, but the saying that warm milk will help you sleep has been around so long that the thought of a warm glass of milk makes me sleepy.

Hair

For healthy hair it is also recommended to eat dark green vegetables. To help your hair grow, salmon, beans (legumes), and avocados are said improve strength and growth of hair. Eggs help with the health of hair. In general, eating good nutritious foods is good for the scalp, hair strength, and growth.

Eyesight

Yes, carrots are good for eyesight. Carrots, squash, and blueberries are all proven to benefit night vision. Eggs, fish, nuts, berries, and dark, leafy vegetables contain nutrients to help with the health of your eyes. All these foods also contain other beneficial nutrients, so even if these foods do not provide results you can see, they should provide results you can feel.

Foods That Lie

One of the first nutritional books I read opened my eyes to the tricks and misleading information that marketers use to sell their products. I couldn't believe that even though their product said 'diet', it was not low calorie. Or that a store claiming to sell health food also has fat-promoting products on their shelves. Diet food and food that is good for your body can be two different things. Luckily we have a nutrition fact label on product packages that are untainted by marketers.

The nutrition fact label might be the only truthful piece of information on the whole package. If a package says fat free, this does not mean it is calorie free. If a package states, 50 calories per serving, check to see how many servings are in the package to get the total calorie content.

Some marketing techniques will take advantage of a small trace of a nutrient in their product and advertise that the whole product is good for you because of this nutrient even though there are other ingredients that are not healthy. While shopping, you might want your foods to take a lie detector test before taking them home with you.

Healthy Fast-food Choices

Do you want fries with that? Fast food restaurants are changing their menus to include more healthy choices. Healthier lifestyles are becoming more and more popular. With the public demand for healthier food, most fast food menu items commonly include grilled chicken breasts and salads. Unfortunately, if you eat a chicken breast with high calorie, high fat sauce on it, you do not lower your calorie intake. If you dump high calorie, high fat dressing on that low calorie salad, you have also cancelled any benefit you could have gained from eating the salad. So how do you find beneficial foods from fast food restaurants? Look for the most simple, identifiable foods that you can find.

Most people think of sandwich restaurants as the healthiest option in fast food. Be aware that many types of bread in sandwich restaurants can hide high calorie content. Tuna fish mixtures sound like they are low calorie, but some contain a high calorie, high fat mayonnaise mix.

The safest and healthiest fast food choices are the ones that are natural and unprocessed. Look for lean meats like chicken, turkey, or fish (not fried). Fried food will add excess calories and fat to your meal.

When servers ask if you want fries and a soda with that, it is as if they are asking you to have extra fat on your butt. Do yourself a favor and say "no." Your health and your butt will thank you for it.

Healthy Eating On A Budget

Many college students are under the impression that the cheap packs of noodles or peanut butter and jelly sandwiches are smart foods. Yes, these are great foods when you are on a budget; however, there are better choices. For example, rice is an inexpensive choice that provides good nutrition and can be mixed with most anything. Beans are another good high nutrition choice that can fit into any budget. Next, you will need some protein to mix into your rice. Chicken, turkey, lean beef, and some kinds of fish are relatively inexpensive (especially on sale).

Oats and eggs are inexpensive staple foods. Make sure to compare fruits and vegetable prices at different stores, some will have better prices than others. Simple salads can be inexpensive to make. To get the most out of your money, make a large quantity, like a large salad or a stew and eat a little at a time through the week.

The dollar menus at fast food restaurants have hardly anything of nutritional value on them. Yes, you get what you pay for. Don't substitute healthy eating for cheap food.

Fat Burning Foods

To burn fat, your metabolism uses food to provide energy for body functions. Some foods and drinks will increase your metabolism rate more than others. First and foremost is water, because every system in your body relies on adequate hydration to work properly; make sure to drink enough water. Green tea, coffee, and low fat milk help to boost metabolism in the body.

Fish, hot peppers, lemon, almonds, eggs, brussel sprouts, celery, cabbage, broccoli, oatmeal, and turkey are all metabolism boosters. Spices such as cinnamon can also contribute to fat burning.

Fiber is another contributor to fat burning by increasing the effectiveness of the digestive system. These foods have high fiber content: grapefruit, berries, lentils, artichokes, and whole grains. Most fruits and vegetables are excellent sources of fiber and contain very few calories.

So if you are planning to cut calories and lose some weight, get some help from these foods. Remember that moderation is key, and overeating fat burning foods (or any foods) will defeat your purpose and cause you to gain weight. Yes, you can gain weight if you eat too much fat burning foods; it doesn't seem fair, I know. So, sensible meals with these foods will put them to work for you, large quantities will put them to work against you.

A Treat Is Not A Treat

You have just got home from a hard day and you don't feel like cooking. You are hungry and after your long day you feel like treating yourself to the greasiest patty on the planet slapped between two buns. Or you step into the local convenience store and decide to treat yourself to a king size candy bar with chocolate on top of chocolate.

You are watching your weight, and you decide to treat yourself and go on a binge at the buffet because you did so well the first part of the week. You will not be doing yourself a favor because unfair as it is, it takes longer to lose weight then it does to put it on, and that one buffet will remove all the hard work you did

There can be nothing wrong with the occasional treat of high calorie foods, it is when it becomes a daily habit then you start feeling the effects that your treat is not a treat to your body or your health. Find your treats with beneficial foods that your body can use, and you will have a win - win situation.

Many people believe that if you have a craving for a certain kind of food, it is your body telling you that you are lacking a certain nutrient that this food possesses. Unfortunately, this has proven not to be the case. It would be nice if cravings did let us know what nutrients we needed; it is most likely that your body wouldn't find the nutrients it was searching for in your ice cream and chocolate cravings anyway.

Losing Weight

There are countless plans and ways to lose weight, most are marketed and usually the creator is more concerned with profit than the public's well-being. I have written a whole book about nutrition and eating without once mentioning the word "diet" until now. This is because I believe that diet is a four-letter word and need not be mentioned anymore.

So what is the correct way to lose weight? The answer is different for everyone, what works for some people may not work for others, but eating good, low calorie, nutritious food will help. How much you should eat depends on many variables like body weight, age, and activity level.

Some weight loss plans take years to see any results. One method that has worked for me, and many others, is to cut portions. I wanted results that I could see and feel fast, so I was advised to cut my portion size in half. When I cut the amount of food at every meal in half, I could see the weight dropping. I don't recommend this method because it is not easy and you feel hungry until you get used to a smaller portion size, but it works.

Other helpful advice that works is to remove all sugary, salty foods and snacks, along with fattening dressings, from your cupboard and refrigerator and stock only healthy food. Use plastic cups and make yourself ready to go snacks by putting fruit and vegetables in them. Find a friend who also wants to lose weight and be each other's support. Add some exercise and say goodbye to unwanted pounds.

Fruits And Vegetables

Fruits and vegetables deserve their own section in this book because of all the benefits that they provide to the body. The rule of thumb is to eat five different colored servings of fruits and vegetables every day; this will ensure your body a wide variety of nutrients. In some countries, fruits and vegetables are main dishes and not just side dishes.

To give your body the best source of nutrients, it is best to consume whole fruits and vegetables as opposed to juices and dried sources. This will ensure that your nutrients are full strength, and not reduced or lost in the processing. A regular diet with a variety of fruits and vegitables can help with endurance by increased blood flow and lung capacity.

Here are some other benefits of fruits and vegetables that you might not know:

- Lemons and limes help to smooth skin.
- Onions can help kill bacteria.
- Apples help improve lung capacity.
- Cabbage helps hemorrhoids.
- Bananas can block diarrhea.
- Carrots can prevent constipation.
- Pineapple dissolves warts.
- Cauliflower can help strengthen bones.

Changing Your Eating Habits

If you haven't guessed it by now, there are some foods you should be eating and some foods you should be eating rarely or avoiding. The closer food is to its natural state, the better it is for the body.

In my opinion, there are five foods that are the best of the best. These foods promote healthy lifestyles. Salmon, blueberries, broccoli, almonds, and green tea have the most powerful health inducing properties.

I wish I could claim that if everyone ate these foods, there would be no more diseases in the world. Because everybody's body is different, it is not possible to make this claim. I can state, with a clear conscience, that there would be *less* sickness and disease in the world if everyone ate healthier foods such as these.

I have not needed to visit a hospital in 25 years, or had to call in sick to work (for reasons of being sick). Having written that, I have most likely jinxed myself and will probably be in the hospital tomorrow. I feel that making the right food choices has made a difference with my health, and I have talked to others who feel that eating the right foods has made positive difference in their life.

Smart Foods

We have smart water, smart phones, and we also have smart foods. Also called super foods, these smart foods provide many benefits to the human body, things like helping you live longer, keeping you from getting sick, and so on. Many of these foods have been listed more than once in this book because of their ability to provide more than one kind of beneficial nutrient. If you regularly eat these foods, you should consider yourself smart.

Here is a list of them: almonds, apples, beans, blueberries, broccoli, green tea, oats, oranges, pumpkin, salmon, soy, tomatoes, turkey, and walnuts are the most well known. With this long a list, everyone is sure to find something that suits their taste. Unfortunately, there is not just one single kind of food that will provide everything that the body needs, so include a good variety of these foods.

I am sorry to disappoint those people hoping to find pastries and candy bars on the list, but they just don't have enough beneficial ingredients. In fact, there were not any nutrition bars that made the list either. So try as we might, Mother Nature still makes the best food on the planet.

Foods That Cleanse

If you have regularly been eating junk foods, or foods that are highly processed, fried, or high in sugar and salt, you could be due for a body cleansing. Cleansing is a natural method to help your body and organs clean your system of toxins and waste.

The cleansing process takes three days and involves drinking water, juices, eating easily digestible foods and herbs. While cleansing, you want to make sure you do not eat processed sugar, fried foods, pasta, beans, eggs, or dairy. If you eat meat, make sure it is lean and in small amounts.

For three days, drink eight to twelve glasses of water per day. Drink two glasses of fruit juice, three glasses of vegetable juice, and three glasses of herbal tea per day. Eat fresh raw fruits and vegetables, seafood, nuts, seeds, and whole grains only.

Cleansing herbs are available from health food stores. Burdock root and dandelion help cleanse toxins from the body.

Now that you have cleaned your body from toxins and junk food, you can feel better if you decide to put toxins and junk back in. Some people perform the cleansing process once a month.

Food Myths

Here are some popular food myths that you were most likely told or led to believe. Many of these myths were spread by a person who didn't have all of their facts together, then told the myth to other people, who then spread it all over the world.

Myth #1   **Eating celery will burn more calories than you consume by eating it, making it a negative calorie food.** Unfortunately negative calorie foods do not exist, a stalk of celery has very little calories, but more than you burn by chewing it.

Myth #2   **Eating six small meals a day will help you lose weight.** The problem with this myth is that most people do not eat small meals, they end up consuming more calories and do not lose weight. This could be true if the six meals had less calories than three.

Myth #3   **You will gain more weight if you eat meals late at night.** It doesn't matter what time it is. When you consume calories, they are the same calories in the morning or at night.

Myth #4   **You will get cramps if you swim after you eat.** No cramps, your body digests food the same in or out of the water.

Myth #5   **Gum will stay in your stomach for seven year**s. No. If myths were true, I would have several packs of gum in my stomach by now, and a few watermelon trees from swallowing seeds.

Foods In Other Countries

The cuisines and snacks of other countries can be very different than our own, for example, eating insects is common in areas of Thailand. Tradition, religion, and availability are among factors that determine what is eaten in other countries.

The types of food that we eat can be just as different to people in other countries. Just as common as we would eat potato chips or a handful of nuts, a Japanese teenager might snack on a mixture of dried sardines and slivered almonds, or a person in South Africa might enjoy a handful of roasted ants and termites.

Our variety of cheeses is puny when compared to the Italians, who have over 400 different kinds of cheeses. Our spice rack would be very laughable to a person in India. A bottle of olive oil might last a couple months or more in the cabinet of an American family. That same bottle would be gone within a week by a family in Greece.

You might see very few stray dogs in China and Korea because dog can be served over rice. When was the last time you had fried snail? In France, people eat five hundred million snails per year, Yum!

More Food Facts

Food facts of note:

- There is no such thing as the 24-hour flu, it is food poisoning.
- Food can only be tasted if it is mixed with saliva.
- Peanuts are used to manufacture dynamite.
- Apples are members of the rose family.
- Pineapples can weigh up to 20 pounds.

Food facts from the past:

- The first soup was made of hippopotamus.
- Ketchup was sold in 1830 as medicine.
- Popcorn has been around for 6,000 years
- Pumpkins were once recommended to remove freckles.
- Coca-cola was originally green.

Fast food facts

- About half the calories in an average fast food meal is from fat.
- Americans drink over 13 billion gallons of soft drinks each year.
- Americans eat approximately 100 acres of pizza each day.
- In 2006, Americans spent 142 billion on fast food.
- Americans eat 1 million animals an hour.

The Future Of Food

Food in the future will most likely continue the trend and become more and more processed with little to no resemblance to raw food. Additives and preservatives will be the norm. The demand for fast and cheap food from consumers, and high profit margins for manufacturers will have these manufacturers searching for the cheapest ingredients to produce their food.

Marketers paid on a commission basis of how well they can sell a product will be more concerned about the company's bottom line dollar and less concerned about the health content of the product they are selling. Stores selling these products will place their most profitable food products, regardless of nutritional content, in the front of the store to have the most visibility to the consumer.

Even though this process is already taking place, we as consumers control the food market, not the manufacturers. If we stop buying foods that do not provide benefits to the body, manufacturers will change the products they make.

We as consumers, have the ability to control the future of food and our health. Retailers such as organic foods stores and farmers markets specialize in unprocessed whole foods that contain the most nutrients. If you want full control over the foods you eat, start a garden, or have neighbors chip in and start a neighborhood garden.

Be Your B-E-S-T

Every person wants to look and feel the best that they possibly can. The human body has some basic requirements to be able to accomplish this goal. This is called being your **BEST**.

B -	**Be active**
E -	**Eat good food**
S -	**Sleep well**
T -	**Think positive**

These are the most basic steps to good health, but they are also the most overlooked. Being active has been proven to keep your physical and mental wellbeing in balance. Include daily physical exercise into your schedule. Eat good, nutritious food that your body can use. Stay away from, or limit, your junk food intake; your body will thank you for it. Sleep well, and enough to recharge your body and mind. Think positive. Dwelling on negative thoughts can deteriorate your physical and mental well-being. Making sure to take these steps daily will ensure that you can look and feel your BEST.

Students preparing for a test, athletes getting ready for a competition, an interviewee interviewing for a job, all must be at their BEST. It can be quite obvious to tell if a person is not at their BEST, their performance will speak for itself. If you miss even one of these steps, it will show.

Checklist

Here is a basic checklist for daily healthy eating tips.

- Drink water
- Eat five different fruit servings per day.
- Eat five different vegetable servings per day.
- Eat lean meats.
- Eat whole grains

Foods you should eliminate or minimize include:

- Fried foods
- Sweets
- Excess salts
- Excess sugars
- Saturated fats

Final Thought

We live in a world full of choices. There are more bad food choices than good, and being educated about how foods affect your body will help you make the right decision when shopping and eating. If you have a specific goal for your health make sure to choose the foods that lead you towards that goal and not away from it. In a nutshell; to have good health, eat good food.

Resources

The resources used for **The Educated Eating Manual** came from nutrition web sites, health books, my own personal experiences, and the experiences of others.

In putting together the manual, I found that doctors and nutrition experts didn't always see eye to eye. Some experts believed one fact, and others believed something else. In cases like this, I was guided by majority opinion and my own experience.

About The Author

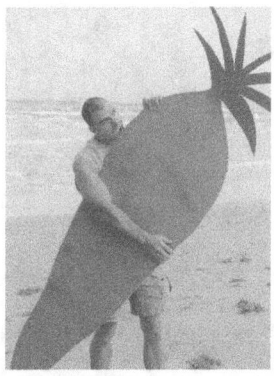

Being involved in many different sports, Chris Barrows has always been interested in ways to increase his body's performance. Looking for informational sources to provide answers, he found that there was not one source that supplied all the information. Chris began writing **The Educated Eating Manual** after finding foods that have kept him from getting sick and put him in the best shape of his life, with the hopes that it will do the same for others.

Chris currently lives, works, and plays on Padre Island, Corpus Christi, Texas

www.ingramcontent.com/pod-product-compliance
Lightning Source LLC
Chambersburg PA
CBHW071300280526
45788CB00004B/1792